10 Minute

CHAIR YOGA

20-Day Beginner, Intermediate And Advanced Challenge To Improve Posture, Mobility, And Heart Health, As Well As Lose Weight.

JOSH L. BUTLER

10 Minute Chair Yoga for Seniors Over 60

20-Day Beginner, Intermediate And Advanced Challenge To Improve Posture, Mobility, And Heart Health, As Well As Lose Weight.

By

Josh L Butler

In the domain of writing, imagination flourishes under the assurance of copyright. This book digs into the legalities shielding the composed universe of **Josh L Butler**. We'll investigate how copyright engages **Josh L Butler** and guarantees her works are delighted in capably.

Disclaimer: This book is for enlightening purposes just and doesn't comprise legitimate counsel.

Table of Content

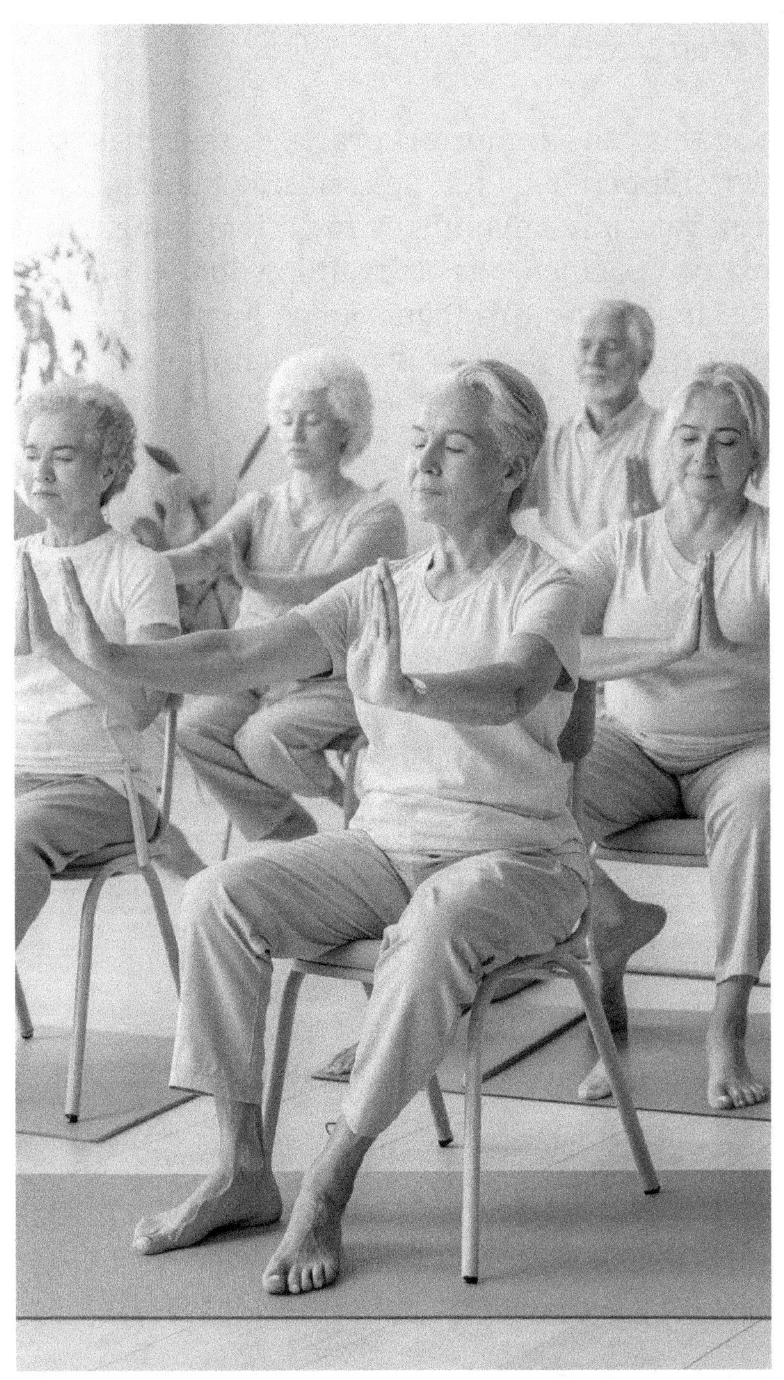

Introduction:

Yoga is an immortal practice that has been worshipped for its physical, mental, and otherworldly advantages for a long time. While many imagine yoga as training done on a mat, its flexibility stretches out a long way past that. In this book, we acquaint you with the awesome universe of seat yoga, explicitly custom-made for seniors north of 60.

Seat yoga offers a delicate yet successful method for encountering the delights of yoga without the requirement for confounded presents or demanding developments. It is open to people of all wellness levels and can be rehearsed anyplace, making it ideal for seniors who might have portability constraints or favor a situated practice.

All through this book, we will investigate a progression of straightforward yet strong seat yoga postures and methods intended to advance adaptability, strength, equilibrium, and unwinding. Whether you're new to yoga or have been rehearsing for quite a long time, these 10-minute seat yoga schedules are ideal for incorporating into your day-to-day practice to upgrade your general prosperity.

Go along with us on this excursion as we find the groundbreaking force of seat yoga and set out on a way to more noteworthy well-being, imperativeness, and internal harmony. We should start our training together, each breath in turn.

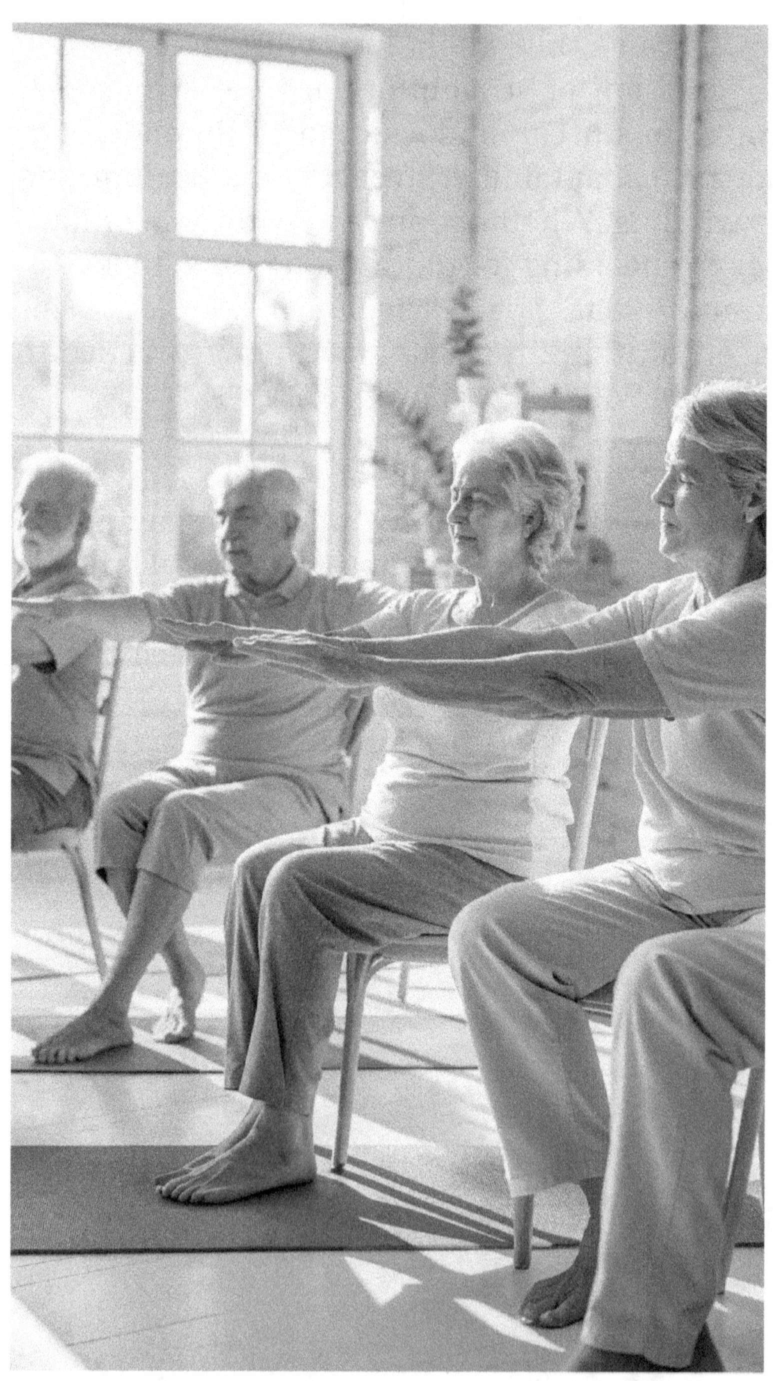

Seat yoga, as the name proposes, is a changed type of yoga that is drilled while situated on a seat or involving a seat for help. It offers a delicate way to deal with yoga, making it open to people of any age and wellness level, especially seniors beyond 60 years old. In this complete clarification, we will dive into the beginnings, advantages, methods, and contemplations of seat yoga.

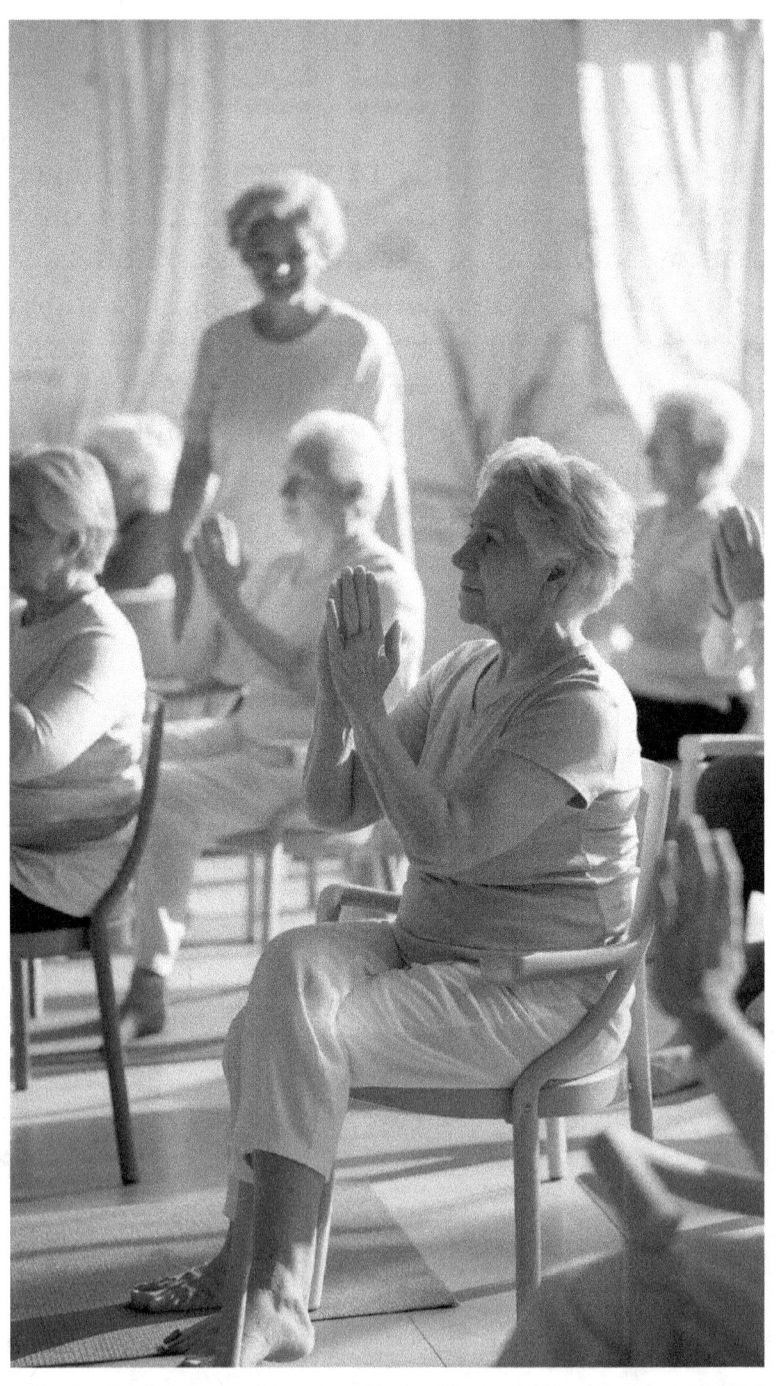

Starting points of Seat Yoga:

Seat yoga follows its underlying foundations back to the customary act of Hatha yoga, which began in old India. While conventional yoga includes standing, situated, and resting presents on a mat, seat yoga arose as a variety to oblige people with actual limits or portability issues. It was at first evolved to give remedial advantages to seniors, people with inabilities, or those recuperating from wounds.

Advantages of Seat Yoga:

Further developed Adaptability: Seat yoga advances delicate extending of the muscles, ligaments, and tendons, upgrading adaptability and scope of movement. This is especially helpful for seniors who might encounter solidness or joint uneasiness.

Improved Strength: Despite being situated, seat yoga consolidates different represents that draw in and reinforce different muscle gatherings, including the center, arms, legs, and back. Developing fortitude is fundamental for keeping up with practical autonomy and forestalling falls in more established grown-ups.

Better Equilibrium and Strength: Many seat yoga poses center around further developing equilibrium and steadiness by focusing on the center muscles and rehearsing care. Upgraded balance diminishes the gamble of falls, which is a typical worry among seniors.

Stress Decrease: Seat yoga underscores profound breathing, unwinding procedures, and care rehearses, which assist with diminishing pressure, uneasiness, and strain. This can add to work on mental prosperity and personal satisfaction.

Torment The board: A normal act of seat yoga can lighten persistent agony related to conditions like joint inflammation, back torment, and fibromyalgia. Delicate development and extension assist with delivering strain in the muscles and advance dissemination, prompting relief from discomfort and expanded solace.

Mind-Body Association: Seat yoga urges members to zero in on their breath, and body sensations, and present second mindfulness. This cultivates a more profound association between the psyche and body, advancing by and large concordance and equilibrium.

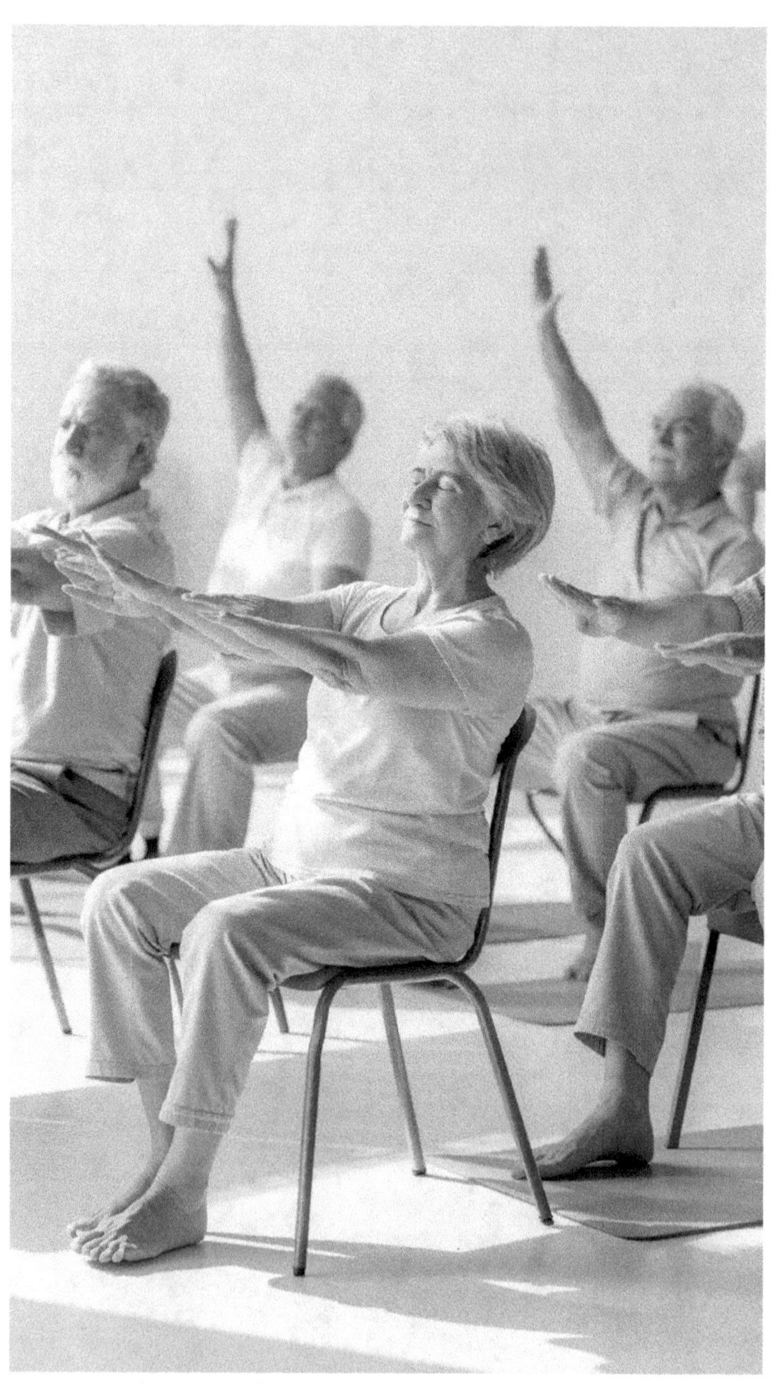

Methods and Practices:

Seat yoga incorporates a great many procedures and practices that can be customized to individual necessities and inclinations. A few normal components of seat

Yoga include:

Situated Represents: These are yoga representations that can be performed while situated on a seat, zeroing in on extending and reinforcing different muscle gatherings. Models incorporate situated ahead twists, spinal winds, and side stretches.

Breathing Activities: Seat yoga integrates breathing procedures, for example, profound diaphragmatic breathing, substitute nostril breathing, and careful relaxing. Cognizant breathing aides quiet the psyche, lessen pressure, and stimulate the body.

Care Contemplation: Reflection is a central part of yoga that develops mindfulness, presence, and inward harmony. Seat yoga frequently incorporates directed contemplation or perception practices to advance unwinding and mental lucidity.

Unwinding Methods: Seat yoga meetings commonly end with a time of unwinding, during which members are urged to rest profoundly and discharge pressure from the body and brain. This might include directed unwinding scripts, moderate muscle unwinding, or representation works out.

Contemplations for seniors:

While rehearsing seat yoga, seniors ought to remember the accompanying contemplations to guarantee a protected and pleasant experience:

Stand by listening to Your Body: Focus on how your body feels during each posture and adjust depending on the situation to keep away from strain or inconvenience. Honor your limits and just go similarly as feels great for you.

Use Props for Help: Seats, pads, blocks, and lashes can be utilized to adjust presents and offer extra help or security. Use props on a case-by-case basis to adjust the training to your interesting requirements.

Remain Hydrated: Drink a lot of water previously, during, and after your seat yoga practice to remain hydrated and support your body's normal capabilities.

Counsel you're Medical Services Supplier: If you have any clinical worries or previous medical issues, talk with your medical care supplier before beginning another activity program, including seat yoga.

Practice Routinely: Consistency is vital to encountering the full advantages of seat yoga. Expect to integrate seat yoga into your everyday daily schedule, regardless of whether it's only for a couple of moments every day.

Seat yoga is a delicate yet strong practice that offers various physical, mental, and close-to-home advantages for seniors older than 60. By making yoga open and comprehensive, seat yoga enables people to work on their general well-being and prosperity, paying little heed to mature or actual restrictions. Whether you're hoping to increment adaptability, diminish pressure, or essentially partake in a snapshot of unwinding, seat yoga gives an inviting space to all to investigate the groundbreaking force of yoga. Embrace the excursion, and may your seat yoga work to give you more noteworthy pleasure, imperativeness, and concordance in your life.

Seat yoga has arisen as a famous and open type of activity and unwinding for seniors north of 60. While customary yoga is frequently connected with complex stances and thorough active work, seat yoga offers a delicate elective that can be rehearsed by people with differing levels of portability and wellness. In this exhaustive investigation, we will dive into the horde of help that seat yoga offers to seniors, enveloping actual well-being, mental prosperity, and close-to-home equilibrium.

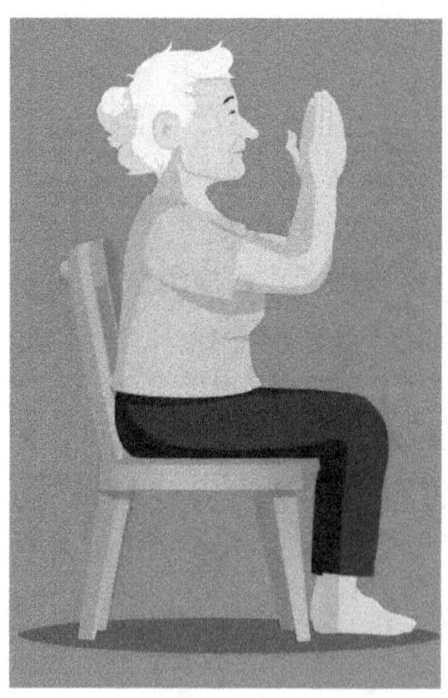

Actual Advantages:

Further developed Adaptability: Seat yoga integrates delicate extending practices that target muscles and joints all through the body. Customary practice can upgrade adaptability, making it simpler for seniors to perform day-to-day exercises like twisting, coming to, and turning.

Improved Strength: Despite being situated, seat yoga connects with different muscle gatherings, including the center, arms, legs, and back. Reinforcing these muscles is critical for keeping up with equilibrium, solidness, and practical freedom as senior's age.

Better Stance: Many seat yoga presents center on spinal arrangement and stance mindfulness, assisting seniors with keeping up with legitimate arrangement and ease issues, for example, slumping or adjusted shoulders. Further developed stance can decrease stress on the spine and forestall normal age-related conditions like kyphosis.

Expanded Scope of Movement: Seat yoga urges seniors to move their bodies through a full scope of movement, which can assist with reducing firmness and joint agony. By tenderly extending and activating the joints, seniors can keep up with or even work on their scope of movement after some time.

Equilibrium and Dependability: Equilibrium is a vital worry for seniors, as falls can prompt serious wounds and loss of freedom. Seat yoga consolidates postures and activities that further develop equilibrium, coordination, and proprioception, decreasing the gamble of falls and upgrading by and large soundness.

Torment The board: Numerous seniors experience constant agony because of conditions like joint inflammation, osteoporosis, or back torment. Seat yoga offers delicate development and extension that can ease torment and distress, advancing more prominent solace and versatility.

Mental and Close-to-Home Advantages:

Stress Decrease: Seat yoga underlines profound breathing, unwinding methods, and care rehearses that assist seniors with diminishing pressure and uneasiness. By zeroing in on the current second and developing a feeling of inward quiet, seniors can more readily deal with the stressors of day-to-day existence.

Further developed State of mind: Actual work, including seat yoga, has been displayed to support temperament and mitigate side effects of misery and uneasiness. The delicate developments and thoughtful parts of seat yoga can elevate spirits and advance a feeling of prosperity in seniors.

Upgraded Mental Capability: Standard activity, for example, seat yoga, has been connected to working on mental capability and memory in more seasoned grown-ups. The psyche-body association encouraged by seat yoga might uphold cerebrum well-being and mental flexibility as senior's age.

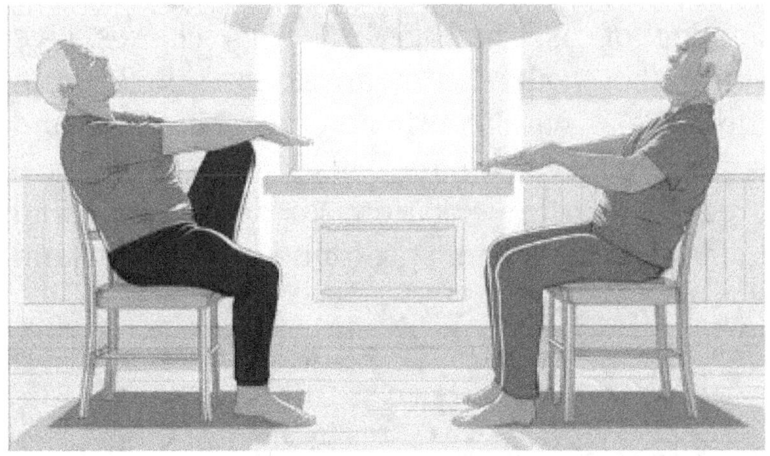

Better Rest: Numerous seniors battle with rest aggravations or sleep deprivation, which can adversely affect by and large well-being and personal satisfaction. Seat yoga advances unwinding and stress alleviation, helping seniors loosen up and get ready for relaxing rest.

Expanded Energy Levels: Regardless of its delicate nature, seat yoga can animate the body and brain, leaving seniors feeling more empowered and alert. Normal practice can further develop flow, invigorate the sensory system, and improve by and large imperativeness.

Feeling of Association: Seat yoga classes give seniors a valuable chance to mingle and interface with others in a strong and comprehensive climate. This feeling of the local area can battle sensations of detachment and dejection, advancing profound prosperity and flexibility.

All-encompassing Advantages:

Mindfulness: Seat yoga urges seniors to tune into their bodies, sensations, and breath, encouraging a more profound identity mindfulness, and self-sympathy. This care practice can prompt more noteworthy acknowledgment and enthusiasm for oneself.

Strengthening: Seat yoga engages seniors to assume command over their well-being and prosperity by furnishing them with apparatuses and methods to help their physical, mental, and close-to-home well-being. Seniors can become dynamic members in their own consideration and mending process.

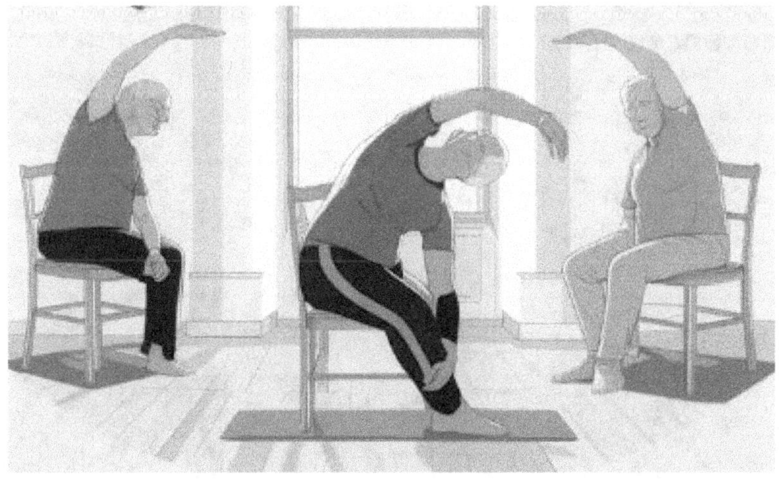

Versatility: One of the best qualities of seat yoga is its flexibility to individual requirements and capacities. Postures can be changed or altered to oblige seniors with fluctuating degrees of versatility, adaptability, or strength, guaranteeing that everybody can take an interest and experience the advantages of yoga.

Long haul Wellbeing: Seat yoga offers seniors a reasonable and pleasant method for keeping up with their well-being and essentialness as they age. Dissimilar to additional difficult types of activity, seat yoga is delicate on the joints and can be drilled securely and easily well into advanced age.

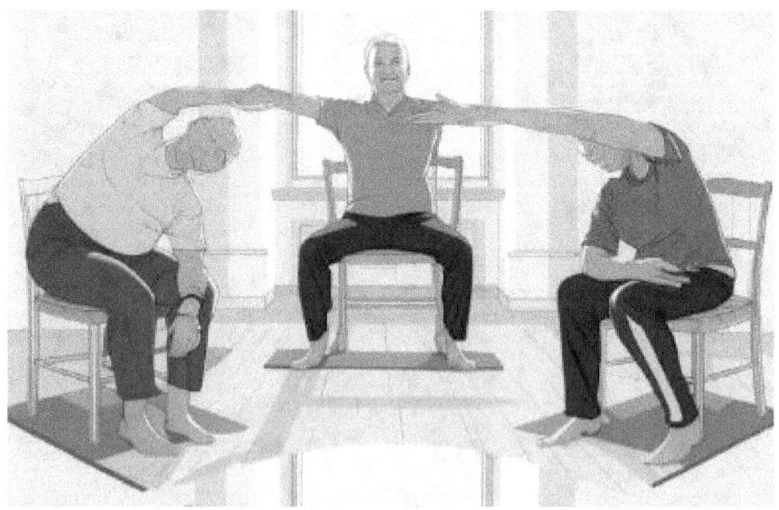

All in all, seat yoga offers an abundance of advantages for seniors older than 60, enveloping actual well-being, mental prosperity, and close-to-home equilibrium. By integrating delicate development, care practices, and unwinding strategies, seat yoga enables seniors to improve their general personal satisfaction and mature smoothly with effortlessness and respect. Whether you're hoping to further develop adaptability, oversee pressure, or essentially partake in a snapshot of harmony, seat yoga gives an inviting space to seniors to investigate the extraordinary force of yoga.

Chapter 3: The Vital Importance of Regular Movement for Older Adults

As people age, keeping up with actual well-being and versatility turns out to be progressively significant for general prosperity and personal satisfaction. Standard development and exercise assume an essential part in advancing life span, freedom, and imperativeness in more established grown-ups. In this far-reaching investigation, we will dive into the complex significance of customary development for seniors, enveloping actual well-being, mental prosperity, and social commitment.

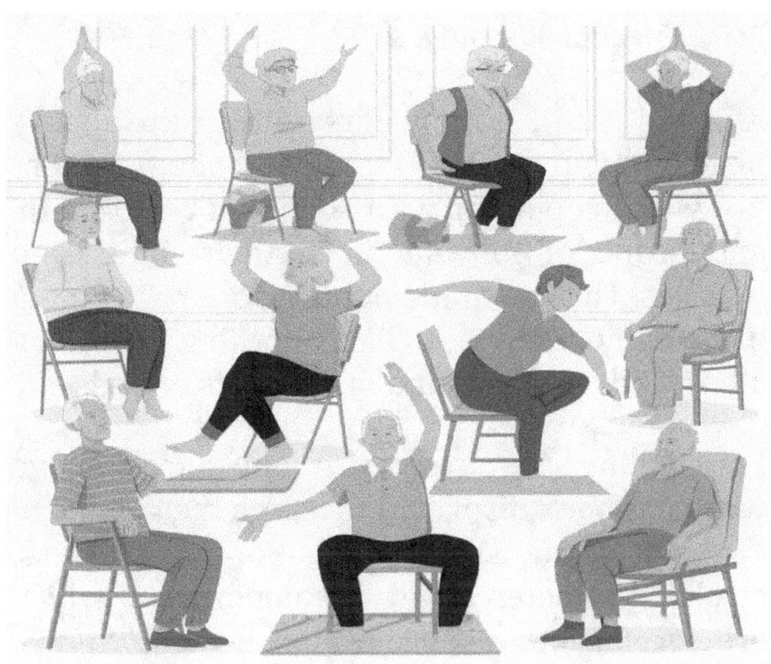

Keeping up with Versatility: Customary development assists more seasoned grown-ups with keeping up with adaptability, strength, and scope of movement in their joints and muscles. This is fundamental for performing day-to-day exercises like strolling, climbing steps, and getting in and out of seats or beds.

Forestalling Persistent Circumstances: Active work has been displayed to lessen the gamble of constant circumstances like coronary illness, stroke, diabetes, and osteoporosis, which are normal among more established grown-ups. The practice assists control of blood pressure, cholesterol levels, and glucose levels, advancing by and large cardiovascular well-being.

Overseeing Weight: As digestion normally eases back with age, keeping a solid weight turns out to be more trying for seniors. Ordinary development, joined with a reasonable eating routine, assists more seasoned grown-ups with overseeing weight and forestalling heftiness-related medical problems like joint torment, joint inflammation, and metabolic disorders.

Further developing Equilibrium and Coordination: Falls are a main source of injury and handicap in more seasoned grown-ups. Ordinary development exercises, including balance activities and strength preparation, assist with further developing equilibrium, coordination, and proprioception, diminishing the gamble of falls and upgrading generally speaking soundness.

Supporting Bone Wellbeing: Weight-bearing activities, like strolling, moving, and opposition preparing, assist with animating bone development and thickness, decreasing the gamble of osteoporosis and breaks. Solid bones are fundamental for keeping up with portability and freedom as senior's age.

Improving Invulnerable Capability: Customary actual work helps the safe framework, lessening the gamble of contaminations and ailments. Practice helps increment dissemination, advance lymphatic seepage, and invigorate the development of invulnerable cells, upgrading the body's capacity to fend off microbes.

Mental Prosperity Advantages:

Lessening Pressure and Tension: Exercise has been displayed to diminish levels of pressure chemicals like cortisol and adrenaline, advancing a feeling of quiet and unwinding. Active work likewise invigorates the arrival of endorphins, synapses that hoist mindsets and lessen sensations of tension and sadness.

Working on Mental Capability: Normal development has been connected to working on mental capability, memory, and leadership capability in more seasoned grown-ups. Practice advances brain adaptability, the cerebrum's capacity to adjust and shape new associations, prompting improved mental versatility and mind well-being.

Upgrading Rest Quality: Actual work can further develop rest quality and span in more seasoned grown-ups, prompting better general rest cleanliness and daytime sharpness. Practice manages circadian rhythms, decreases sleep deprivation side effects, and advances further, more supportive rest.

Helping Confidence and Certainty: Taking part in customary development exercises encourages a feeling of achievement, dominance, and fearlessness in more established grown-ups. Accomplishing wellness objectives, beating actual difficulties, and encountering enhancements in strength and versatility add to a positive mental self-portrait and more prominent confidence.

Mitigating Side Effects of Melancholy: Exercise has been demonstrated to be a powerful adjunctive treatment for sorrow in more established grown-ups. Actual work invigorates the creation of synapses, for example, serotonin and dopamine, which assume a key part in managing state of mind and feelings.

Social Commitment Advantages:

Encouraging Social Associations: Partaking in bunch practice classes, strolling gatherings, or sporting exercises gives amazing open doors to more established grown-ups to mingle, cooperate, and fabricate significant connections. Social commitment is imperative for mental and close-to-home prosperity, especially in later life.

Advancing People Group Consideration: Normal development exercises assist more seasoned grown-ups with feeling associated with their networks and taking part in shared interests and pursuits. Taking part in neighborhood occasions, workout regimes, or open-air exercises cultivates a feeling of having a place and kinship among seniors.

Offering Close-to-Home Help: Gathering exercise settings establish a strong climate where more seasoned grown-ups can energize, spur, and rouse each other. Sharing shared objectives, encounters, and difficulties assists seniors with feeling comprehended, approved, and upheld in their wellness process.

Improving Personal satisfaction: Social communication and significant associations add to a better of life and are more prominent in general fulfillment in more established grown-ups. Normal development exercises give open doors to chuckling, fellowship, and satisfaction, improving seniors' lives in significant and significant ways.

All in all, normal development is fundamental for advancing well-being, essentialness, and joy in more established grown-ups. By integrating actual work into their day-to-day routines, seniors can keep up with versatility, forestall ongoing circumstances, improve mental prosperity, and encourage social associations. Whether it's strolling, swimming, moving, or rehearsing yoga, tracking down charming and feasible ways of remaining dynamic is vital to improving with age and partaking in a satisfying and energetic life.

Chapter 4: Getting Started with Chair Yoga for seniors

Seat yoga offers a delicate yet powerful way for seniors to receive the rewards of yoga while situated easily in a seat or involving a seat for help. Whether you're new to yoga or searching for a changed practice that obliges your versatility needs, seat yoga gives an inviting passage highlighting the groundbreaking universe of yoga. In this complete aid, we will investigate all that you want to be aware of to get everything rolling with seat yoga, including picking the right seat, security precautionary measures, and establishing a loosening up climate for your training.

Figuring out Seat Yoga:

Seat yoga is a changed type of yoga that adjusts customary yoga postures and procedures for people who might experience issues getting on or off the floor or have restricted versatility because of old enough, injury, or incapacity. By using a seat for help, solidness, and equilibrium, seat yoga permits members to encounter the advantages of yoga without the requirement for complex mat-based presents or demanding developments.

Advantages of Seat Yoga:

Further developed Adaptability: Seat yoga consolidates delicate extending practices that assist with further developing adaptability, scope of movement, and joint versatility, making it simpler to perform everyday exercises effortlessly and with solace.

Upgraded Strength: Regardless of being situated, seat yoga draws in different muscle gatherings, including the center, arms, legs, and back, advancing strength, steadiness, and practical freedom in seniors.

Better Equilibrium and Steadiness: Seat yoga remembers postures and activities that concentrate on further developing equilibrium, coordination, and proprioception, diminishing the gamble of falls and upgrading generally speaking soundness in more seasoned grown-ups.

Stress Decrease: Seat yoga underlines profound breathing, unwinding procedures, and care rehearses that assist with diminishing pressure, uneasiness, and strain, advancing a feeling of quiet and inward harmony.

Torment the executives: Seat yoga can lighten ongoing agony related to conditions like joint pain, back torment, and fibromyalgia by tenderly extending and activating the muscles and joints, prompting expanded solace and prosperity.

Picking the Right Seat:

Select a solid, stable seat without wheels, armrests that are not excessively wide, and a seat that is level and level.

Guarantee that the seat is the right level for you, permitting your feet to lay serenely on the floor with your knees twisted at a 90-degree point.

Security Safeguards:

Talk with your medical services supplier before beginning another activity program, including seat yoga, particularly on the off chance that you have any ailments or actual impediments.

Pay attention to your body and try not to drive yourself into represents that cause agony or distress. Alter acts like expected to suit your singular necessities and capacities.

Use props like pads, blocks, or lashes to help your body and improve strength and solace during your training.

Establishing a Loosening up Climate:

Find a tranquil, sufficiently bright space where you can rehearse seat yoga without interruptions.

Set the state of mind by diminishing the lights, playing delicate music, or lighting candles to make a quiet and peaceful climate.

Dress easily in baggy apparel that considers the opportunity for development and breathability.

Neck Stretches:

Sit easily in your seat with your feet level on the floor and your spine tall.

Delicately slant your head aside, bringing your ear towards your shoulder, and hold for a couple of breaths. Rehash on the opposite side.

Gradually turn your head in a roundabout movement, moving clockwise and afterward counterclockwise, to deliver strain in the neck and shoulders.

Shoulder Rolls:

Breathe in as you lift your shoulders towards your ears, and breathe out as you roll them back and down, crushing your shoulder bones together.

Rehash this development a few times, switching back and forth between forward and reverse shoulder rolls, to deliver pressure and further develop course in the shoulders.

Profound Breathing Activities:

Sit tall in your seat with your feet level on the floor and your hands lying kneeling.

Breathe in profoundly through your nose, growing your gut and ribcage, and breathe out leisurely through your mouth, delivering any strain or stress.

Rehash this profound breathing activity a few times, zeroing in on the vibe of the breath streaming all through your body.

Situated Ahead Twist (Paschimottanasana):

Sit towards the front edge of your seat with your feet hip-width separated and level on the floor.

Breathe in as you protract your spine, and breathe out as you pivot forward from your hips, bringing your chest towards your thighs.

Clutch the sides of your seat or put your hands on your shins, lower legs, or feet, contingent upon your adaptability.

Loosen up your neck and shoulders, and inhale profoundly into the stretch for a few breaths.

Situated Spinal Turn (Ardha Matsyendrasana):

Sit tall in your seat with your feet level on the floor and your spine stretched.

Breathe in as you extend your spine, and breathe out as you turn your middle to the right, putting your left hand outwardly on your right knee and your right hand on the rear of the seat.

Keep your hips grounded and your shoulders loose as you tenderly wind from the abdomen, investigating your right shoulder.

Hold the contort for a few breaths, then, at that point, return to fixate and rehash on the opposite side.

Situated Feline Cow Stretch:

Sit serenely in your seat with your feet level on the floor and your hands lying kneeling.

Breathe in as you curve your back and lift your chest towards the roof, drawing your shoulder bones together (Cow Posture).

Breathe out as you round your spine and fold your jawline towards your chest, drawing your paunch button towards your spine (Feline Posture).

Stream flawlessly among Feline and Cow Postures, synchronizing your breath with development, for a few rounds.

Profound Unwinding:

Sit back in your seat with your feet level on the floor and your hands lying on your lap.

Shut your eyes and take a few full breaths, permitting your body to unwind.

Discharge any pressure or stress with each breath out, sinking further into a condition of unwinding with every breath.

Stay in this casual state for a few minutes, partaking in the vibes of smoothness and peacefulness.

Getting everything rolling with seat yoga is an enabling excursion that offers innumerable advantages for seniors, including further developed adaptability, strength, equilibrium, and unwinding. By picking the right seat, rehearsing security insurance, and establishing a calming climate for your training, you can leave extraordinarily to more noteworthy well-being and prosperity. Whether you're hoping to ease the strain, increment portability, or essentially partake in a snapshot of harmony, seat yoga gives a delicate yet successful method for feeding your body, brain, and soul. Embrace the excursion, and may your seat yoga work to give you more noteworthy pleasure, imperativeness, and concordance in your life.

Chapter 7: The Importance of Choosing the Right Chair for Chair Yoga Practice

While starting a seat yoga work, choosing the right seat is a basic step towards guaranteeing solace, security, and viability. The seat fills in as a steady and strong base for performing yoga presents, working with legitimate arrangement and simplicity of development. In this exhaustive aid, we will investigate the fundamental variables to consider while picking a seat for seat yoga work, including solidness, size and aspects, materials, and extra elements.

Solidness:

The solidness of the seat is central for protected and powerful seat yoga practice. Search for a seat with a tough edge and strong development that can uphold your weight without wobbling or spilling. Stay away from seats with wheels, as they might be shaky during specific postures and could prompt mishaps or wounds. A seat with non-slip elastic feet or hold cushions on the base can give extra soundness and forestall sliding on smooth surfaces.

Size and Aspects:

Consider the size and aspects of the seat to guarantee an agreeable and obliging practice space. The seat ought to be adequately wide to serenely uphold your hips and consider the opportunity for development without feeling confined or compelled. The seat level ought to be suitable for your body size, permitting your feet to lay level on the floor with your knees bowed at a 90-degree point. Moreover, the backrest level ought to offer sufficient help for your spine without feeling excessively prohibitive or nosy.

Materials:

Pick a seat produced using solid materials that can endure customary use and give dependable solace. Search for seats with padded seats and backrests upholstered in breathable and simple to-clean texture or vinyl. Keep away from seats with hard, awkward seats or unpleasant, scratchy upholstery that might cause uneasiness during delayed use. Furthermore, consider the weight limit of the seat to guarantee it can securely uphold your body weight without compromising steadiness or underlying honesty.

Extra Elements:

A few seats might accompany extra highlights or changes that improve their reasonableness for seat yoga practice. Search for seats with armrests that are not excessively wide or obstructive, taking into consideration the unhindered development of the arms and shoulders. Seats with flexible level or shift instruments can oblige individual inclinations and offer ideal help and arrangement during training. Also, seats with removable or collapsing parts might offer more prominent flexibility and accommodation for capacity and transportation.

Remember that the right seat for seat yoga practice might fluctuate depending on individual requirements, inclinations, and actual restrictions. Consider your particular necessities and any current medical issues or versatility challenges while choosing a seat. Seats with adjustable elements or movable parts can oblige an extensive variety of body types and capacities, making them reasonable for specialists of any age and wellness level.

Before settling on a last choice, get some margin to try out various seats to figure out which one feels generally great and strong for your body. Sit in the seat for a lengthy period to survey its general solace, security, and ergonomic plan. Focus on how your body feels in different situated positions and yoga presents, making changes on a case-by-case basis to guarantee ideal arrangement and simplicity of development.

Picking the right seat is a basic part of laying out a protected, agreeable, and viable seat yoga practice. By focusing on strength, size and aspects, materials, and extra elements, you can choose a seat that meets your particular requirements and upgrades your yoga experience. Whether you're a fledgling or an accomplished specialist, putting resources into a quality seat that upholds your body and lines up with your training objectives is fundamental for expanding the advantages of seat yoga and advancing generally speaking well-being and prosperity. Embrace the excursion, and may your seat yoga work to give you more prominent pleasure, essentialness, and amicability in your life.

Security is foremost while taking part in any type of active work, including seat yoga. While seat yoga is for the most part protected and open for people of any age and wellness level, it's vital to play it safe to forestall wounds and guarantee an agreeable and charming practice insight. In this aide, we will frame key security safeguards to remember while rehearsing seat yoga, incorporating talking with medical care experts, paying attention to your body, and involving props for help.

Talk with Your Medical Services Supplier:

Before beginning another activity program, including seat yoga, it's fundamental to talk with your medical services supplier, particularly assuming that you have any previous ailments or actual restrictions. Your medical services supplier can give customized direction and suggestions given your singular well-being status, guaranteeing that seat yoga is protected and fitting for your requirements.

One of the main security safety measures in seat yoga practice is to pay attention to your body and honor its signs and limits. Focus on how your body feels during each posture and development, and try not to drive yourself into places that cause agony or uneasiness. Recall that yoga isn't tied in with accomplishing a specific degree of adaptability or execution but about interfacing with your body and tracking down straightforwardness and solace in each stance.

Seat yoga postures can be altered or adjusted to suit your one-of-a-kind requirements and capacities. If you experience issues with a specific posture, make sure to do it by utilizing props like pads, blocks, or lashes for help. For instance, on the off chance that you have tight hamstrings, you can put a pad under your hips in situated ahead curves to decrease the burden on the lower back and hamstrings. Be innovative and investigate various changes to find what turns out best for your body.

Props are priceless apparatuses for improving security, solace, and arrangement in seat yoga practice. Try different things by utilizing pads, blocks, lashes, or even collapsed covers to help your body and work on your stance in different postures. Props can assist you with keeping up with appropriate arrangements, forestall overextending or stressing, and make testing presents more available and pleasant. Feel free to props generously to establish a protected and strong practice climate.

While it's vital to challenge yourself and investigate your edge-in-seat yoga practice, it's similarly critical to keep away from overexertion and propelling yourself excessively hard. Find a steady speed during your training and enjoy reprieves depending on the situation to rest and re-energize. Recollect that seat yoga is about delicate, careful development and unwinding, not tied in with driving yourself as far as possible or compelling your body into awkward positions.

Remain Hydrated:

Keeping up with legitimate hydration is fundamental for supporting your body's regular capabilities and forestalling drying out during seat yoga practice. Make certain to drink a lot of water previously, during, and after your training meeting, particularly if you're rehearsing in a warm or sticky climate. Pay attention to your body's thirst signs and taste water consistently to remain hydrated and empowered all through your training.

Practice Careful Relaxing:

Careful breathing is a critical part of seat yoga practice and can assist with advancing unwinding, decreasing pressure, and improving concentration and fixation. Focus on your breath as you travel through each posture, breathing in profoundly through your nose and breathing out leisurely through your mouth. Permit your breath to direct your developments and make a feeling of straightforwardness and stream in your training.

Well-being is fundamental in seat yoga practice, and avoiding potential risk can assist with guaranteeing a protected, agreeable, and pleasant experience for professionals of any age and capacity. By talking with your medical care supplier, paying attention to your body, changing postures on a case-by-case basis, involving props for help, keeping away from overexertion, remaining hydrated, and rehearsing careful breathing, you can establish a protected and steady practice climate that advances in general wellbeing and prosperity. Focus on well-being in your seat yoga practice, and may your process be overflowing with happiness, imperativeness, and harmony.

The climate where you practice seat yoga plays a huge part in improving unwinding, concentration, and by and large satisfaction. By making a peaceful and welcoming space, you can improve your training experience and develop a feeling of quiet and prosperity. In this aid, we will investigate useful hints and systems for setting the temperament and establishing a loosening up climate for seat yoga work, including contemplations for lighting, vibe, and tangible components.

Lighting establishes the vibe for your training space and can altogether influence your temperament and energy levels. Go for the gold, lighting that makes a warm and welcoming environment. Normal light is ideal whenever the situation allows, as it gives a delicate, delicate sparkle that advances unwinding and inspires the soul. If rehearsing at night or in a faintly lit room, utilize delicate, movable lighting sources like lights, candles, or string lights to make a comfortable feel. Stay away from unforgiving light fixtures or splendid, glaring lights, as they can be diverting and upset the quieting climate.

Feeling and Style:

The feeling of your training space can enormously impact your perspective and close-to-home prosperity. Pick style and goods that bring out a feeling of peacefulness, concordance, and equilibrium. Consider integrating components of nature, like pruned plants, blossoms, or regular materials like wood or stone, to bring a hint of the outside inside. Delicate, mitigating colors like pastels or earth tones can make a quieting scenery for your training, while fine art or stylistic layouts with moving or peaceful subjects can elevate and motivate you during your training meeting.

Drawing in the faculties can develop your association with your training and improve unwinding and care. Try different things by integrating tangible components like calming music, fragrant healing, or material surfaces into your training space. Pick delicate, instrumental music or nature sounds that advance unwinding and center, keeping away from anything excessively noisy or diverting. Fragrant healing can be accomplished by utilizing rejuvenating oils, incense, or scented candles with quieting aromas like lavender, chamomile, or sandalwood. You can likewise integrate material components like delicate covers, pads, or finished mats to give solace and establishment during your training.

A messiness-free climate can advance a feeling of quiet and lucidity, permitting you to zero in completely on your training without interruptions. Before beginning your seat yoga meeting, take a couple of seconds to clean up and improve on your training space. Gather up any superfluous things or mess from the area, keeping just the fundamentals reachable. Make a feeling of extensive size and transparency in your training space, considering free development and streaming during your training.

Customize Your Space:

Make your training space your own by customizing it with significant articles, photographs, or keepsakes that give you pleasure and motivation. Encircle yourself with things that inspire and uphold your training, whether it's a most loved statement, a treasured photograph, or an extraordinary piece of work of art. Making a space that mirrors your character and inclinations can improve your association with your training and develop your feeling of presence and care.

Establishing a loosening-up climate for seat yoga practice is fundamental for advancing unwinding, concentration, and in general prosperity. By taking into account factors like lighting, mood, tactile components, cleaning up, and personalization, you can develop a tranquil and welcoming space that improves your training experience and supports your excursion towards more noteworthy well-being and essentialness. Carve out the opportunity to make a training space that sustains your body, brain, and soul, and May your seat yoga practice be loaded up with harmony, bliss, and internal congruity.

Chapter 10: Warm-Up Postures and Neck Stretches

Before jumping into any yoga meeting, it's fundamental to set up the body and brain for certain delicate warm-up presents and stretches. These assist in relaxing tight muscles, expanding blood flow, and upgrading adaptability. Start by sitting easily in a leg-over leg position on your yoga mat.

Neck Stretches:

Delicately slant your head aside, bringing your ear towards your shoulder, feeling a stretch along the opposite side of your neck. Hold for a couple of breaths, then change to the opposite side. Rehash this stretch a couple of times, moving gradually and carefully.

Shoulder Rolls:

Breathe in as you lift your shoulders towards your ears, breathe out as you roll them back and down. Rehash this movement a couple of times, permitting any pressure in your shoulders to soften away with each roll.

Delicate Arm Circles:

Stretch your arms out to the sides at shoulder level. Start making little circles with your arms, continuously expanding the size of the circles as you relax. After a couple of rounds, switch the bearing of the circles.

Profound Breathing Activities:

Shut your eyes and take a couple of full breaths, zeroing in on filling your lungs with each breath in and delivering any strain with each breathe out. This assists with quieting the brain and getting ready for the training ahead.

Situated Asanas (Yoga Stances)

After heating up, change into situated asanas or yoga presents. These can assist with further developing stance, increment adaptability, and developing care.

Situated Ahead Curve (Paschimottanasana):

Expand your legs out before you, flexing your feet towards you. Breathe in to stretch your spine, then breathe out as you pivot forward from your hips, coming towards your toes. Keep your back straight and try not to adjust your spine. Hold for a couple of breaths, then leisurely delivery.

Situated Spinal Turn (Ardha Matsyendrasana):

Get one leg over the other, putting the foot level on the floor. Breathe in to extend your spine, then, at that point, breathe out as you bend towards the bowed knee, putting the opposite hand outwardly of the thigh for help and the other hand behind you. Hold the turn for a couple of breaths, then, at that point, rehash on the opposite side.

Situated Feline Cow Stretch:

Put your hands kneeling. Breathe in as you curve your back, lifting your chest and looking towards the roof (Cow Posture). Breathe out as you round your spine, tucking your jawline towards your chest (Feline Posture). Keep streaming between these two postures with your breath for a few rounds.

Situated Side Stretch:

Expand one arm above, coming towards the contrary side. Keep the two hips grounded as you protract through the side body. Hold for a couple of breaths, then, at that point, switch sides.

Equilibrium and Dependability Stances

Presently, we should zero in on equilibrium and dependability, which are vital for general strength and coordination.

Situated Mountain Posture (Tadasana):

Sit tall with your feet level on the floor and your hands lying on your thighs. Connect with your center and extend through your spine, envisioning yourself as a tall mountain attached to the earth.

Situated Tree Posture (Vrksasana):

Carry the bottom of one foot to lay on the internal thigh or calf of the contrary leg, tracking down your equilibrium. Press your foot into your thigh and your thigh into your foot, feeling a feeling of steadiness and lift through your spine. Hold for a couple of breaths, then, at that point, switch sides.

Situated Leg Lifts:

Broaden one leg out before you, flexing your foot. Breathe in to protract your spine, then, at that point, breathe out as you lift the lengthy leg off the floor, connecting with your center. Hold for a couple of breaths, then, at that point, bring down the leg with control. Rehash on the opposite side.

Unwinding and Contemplation

As we close the training, it's fundamental to require investment for unwinding and contemplation to incorporate the advantages of the training and develop a feeling of internal harmony.

Directed Unwinding Strategies:

Rests on your back in Carcass Posture (Savasana). Shut your eyes and carry attention to each piece of your body, intentionally delivering any strain you might clutch. You can likewise picture a tranquil scene or rehash a quiet mantra to help unwind further.

Care Reflection:

Sit serenely with your eyes shut and carry your thoughtfulness regarding your breath. Notice the impression of each breath in and breathe out, without attempting to change anything. At the point when your brain meanders, tenderly take it back to the breath.

Perception Activities:

Envision yourself in a quiet regular setting, like a lavish woods or a peaceful ocean side. Connect every one of your faculties as you envision the sights, sounds, scents, and impressions of this quiet spot. Permit yourself to feel submerged in the experience.

Shutting and End

As we reach the finish of our training, pause for a minute to ponder how you feel genuinely, intellectually, and inwardly. Recognize any sensations or experiences that emerged during the training, and convey this mindfulness with you as you travel through the remainder of your day.

Cool-Down Stretches:

Get done with some delicate stretches to deliver any leftover pressure in your body. You can return to a portion of the warm-up presents or consolidate other stretches that vibe great for you.

Pondering the Training:

Consider journaling about your experience or just taking a couple of seconds to quietly reflect. Notice any progressions in your mindset, energy levels, or outlook in the wake of finishing the training.

Consolation for Standard Practice:

Help yourself to remember the advantages of a steady yoga practice, both on and off the mat. Focus on setting aside a few minutes for taking care of oneself and care routinely, realizing that each training adds to your general prosperity.

Search out books, recordings, or classes to extend your comprehension and practice of yoga. There are innumerable assets accessible, so investigate and find what impacts you.

Integrating these components into your yoga practice can assist you with developing equilibrium, strength, adaptability, and inward harmony. Make sure to pay attention to your body and honor its necessities as you investigate each posture and reflection procedure. With ordinary practice and persistence, you'll keep on advancing on your excursion towards comprehensive well-being.

THE END.

www.ingramcontent.com/pod-product-compliance
Lightning Source LLC
Chambersburg PA
CBHW050825250726
48653CB00006B/2429